I0463504

Diagnosis and Management of Nightmares and Sleep Disorders in a Jail or Prison Setting.
The long view. Your 41st Consultation
Copyright applied for November 5th, 2023.
William R. Yee M.D., J.D.

ISBN
978-1-304-81167-7

Prologue:

I usually work in an acute care setting that involves unstable individuals with mental illness, drug addiction, homelessness, and severe psychosocial disabilities manifesting symptoms including, but not limited to:

1. suicidal
2. homicidal
3. grave disability
4. severe distress
5. withdrawing from fentanyl
6. withdrawing from methamphetamine
7. withdrawing from alcohol

The mental health team at many facilities approach me regarding clients with nightmares.

Mental illness is not a flat line. There are ups and downs with remissions and exacerbations, without an X-ray or Blood test convenient for determining where they are at any given time.

I am accustomed to working with clients on
1. Poly Pharmacy
2. Poly Addiction
3. Poly Diagnosis
4. Poly Stressors
5. Complicated by
6. Malingering
7. Ganser's Syndrome
8. Factitious Disorders
9. Secondary Gain due to Temporary Insanity
10. Legal Counsel advising clients not to say anything.
11. "I claim the 5th Amendment Right to Silence."
12. "I want to talk to my attorney."

For many reasons as described above and below, my first inclination is to take clients off all medications to determine what the current baseline is for their mental illness.

I find that the mental health team, on the other hand, are inclined to press for an immediate medication for an immediate resolution of symptoms.

As regards immediate medications.

I recommend CIWA lorazepam to prevent withdrawal seizures despite the risk of paradoxical agitation and aggression.

I recommend PO or IM Olanzapine due to its neutral effect on QTc as many psychotropics and substance abuse, including, but not limited to:
1. Alcohol cardiomyopathy – a known cause of Long QTC
2. Methamphetamine– a known cause of Long QTC
3. And Fentanyl– a known cause of Long QTC

The most effective and safest strategy is to treat alcohol withdrawal by CIWA.
1. lorazepam is administered,
2. according to blood pressure,
3. according to pulse,
4. according to temperature,
5. and clients are monitored for seizures and other emergent medical conditions,
6. olanzapine PO or IM is ordered for management of Agitation/Aggression

Stress/Anxiety and Bipolar and Schizophreniform Psychotic Symptoms,

7. clients are monitored for QTc and other heart conditions
8. Treatment of sleep disorders and other chronic conditions are deferred until the acute psychotic episode remits,
9. the suicidal episode remits,
10. the homicidal episode remits,
11. the greave disability remits,
12. there is time and staff available to do the extensive documentation necessary to diagnose and treat the chronic conditions adequately and effectively based upon a comprehensive diagnosis and treatment plan.

Introduction: Context

The reader is advised that the most important recent research is the following:
A. pharmacotherapy does not change. brain activity or connectivity
B. Psychotherapy alters neural activities and connectivity of
C. regions serving
    1. executive control
    2. emotion regulation

3. dialectical behavior therapy and
4. psychodynamic therapies are the
   most effective.

Hallucination like experiences and
delusions are common in
individuals without psychoses.

Every hallucination, every delusion, and
every paranoia should NOT be treated.

I refer the reader to:
Studying Healthy Psychosis like
Experiences to Improve Illness Prediction
Philip R. Corlett, PhD, Sonia Bansal, PhD
James M. Gold, PhD
Published Online: March 8, 2023,
Special Communication

A. Moral Intuitions
1. I would not want this for myself.
2. Treatment is making my patient
   suffer horribly.
3. There is no good option here.
4. No matter what I do, I don't think my
   patient is going to get better.
5. I have no choice but to use coercion.
6. I feel that we're only making matters
   worse.
7. I would not be surprised if my patient

died this year.

B. Thoughts and feelings like these are Associated with,

1. unease,
2. helplessness,
3. being stuck,

C. are common among mental health care professionals

D. especially those caring for persons,

1. with severe and persistent mental illness (SPMI),

E. Typically, these concerns are,

1. dismissed or,
2. attributed to burnout,
3. lack of training or,
4. lack of experience, or
5. unprofessional pessimism.

F. Examine these thoughts through the lens of moral intuition.

1. with the potential,
2. to improve care,
3. of persons living with SPMI.

G. In some cases the pursuit of rehabilitative goals is futile.

1. some have advocated palliative approaches to mental health care
2. the overarching palliative goal in mental health care is to
   a. maximize quality of life
   b. through harm reduction
   c. relief of suffering

I refer the reader to:
Moral Intuitions About Futility as Prompts
for Evaluating Goals in
Mental Health Care
AMA Journal of Ethics
Published Online: September 1, 2023

The Covid Pandemic has altered physical
and mental health in the general
population that requires this addition to my
prior publication.

Recent advances in MRI's, Genetics, DNA
knowledge, and medical technology in
general require this addition to my prior
publications.

There are ethical issues that impinge on the
practice of psychiatry.

One author asks how a psychiatrist should
conduct himself when:
1. There is limited time for CBT
    motivationally enhanced therapy?
2. Are there significant side effects of
    antipsychotics?
3. The client's cognitive functions
    are impaired.

The author does not provide explicit answers, but merely asks questions that are easily asked but without answers that satisfy anyone.

I refer the reader to:
Should Antipsychotics' Risks Be Accepted by Clinicians on Behalf of Patients to Achieve Benefits of Mitigating Older Adults' Behavioral Symptoms in Short-Staffed Units?
Alex Rollo MD, Jena Kar DO, Uma Suryadevara MD et al?
AMA Journal of Ethics
Published Online: October 1, 2023

A. Mental illness accounts for almost
1. 30% of disease burden
2. among noncommunicable diseases
B. Environmental factors account for approximately
1. 50% of the attributable risk for mental disorder
C. Environmental factors that are shared among groups, such as
    1. urbanicity,
    2. climate and
    3. pollution,
    4. regional socioeconomic status,
    5. shared psychosocial stressors, s
    6. such as the COVID-19 pandemic

7. are less well investigated

I refer the reader to: Addressing Global Environmental Challenges to Mental Health Using Population Neuroscience A Review JAMA Psychiatry Published Online: August 23, 2023

Borderline Personality Disorder
1. No class of psychoactive medication is consistently effective
2. No medications is FDA approved for
   Borderline Personality Disorder
3. Pharmacotherapy is not recommend for Treatment of any core symptom of BPD
   A. marked emotional instability
   B. transient stress-related paranoid
      ideation
4. Functional magnetic resonance imaging studies have convincedly demonstrated
   A. pharmacotherapy does NOT change
      brain activity or connectivity,
   B. Psychotherapy
1. ALTERS neural activities and
2. ALTERS connectivity of regions serving
3. executive control
4. emotion regulation
5. dialectical behavior therapy and
6. psychodynamic therapies are effective.

I rely on:

Review of Borderline Personality Disorder
Falk Leichsenring, DSc; Nikolas Heim, MA, MSc3; Frank Leweke, MD1; et al
JAMA Published Online: February 28, 2023
Review

Having provided the above context, I address the issue of treating nightmares in prisons through the lens of an article published October of 2023.

Nightmares and nightmare disorder in adults
AUTHORS: Rochelle Zak, MDAnoop Karippot, MD, FAASM SECTION EDITOR: Alon Y Avidan, MD, MPH DEPUTY EDITORS: April F Eichler, MD, MPH Michael Friedman, MD
All topics are updated as new evidence becomes available and our peer review process is complete.
Literature review current through: Oct 2023.This topic last updated: Oct 18, 2023.

Nightmares are
1. Common
2. beginning early in childhood
3. and extending throughout the lifespan.
4. The condition is strongly associated with
   A. Stress,

B. Anxiety, and
C. trauma.

Nightmares
1. are not by definition pathologic,
2. those that are
3. those that are frequent or disabling and
4. those that are impair social occupational wellbeing
5. those that are impair occupational wellbeing
6. those that are impair emotional well being and
7. those that are impair physical wellbeing
8. are considered a disorder and
9. are often a sign of underlying
10. and treatable psychopathology.

Common causes include.
1. stress,
2. negative life events,
3. the experience of trauma as in
4. posttraumatic stress disorder (PTSD),
5. depression,
6. other psychiatric disorders,
7. +_+_+and medication side effects.+_+_+

This topic reviews the
1. Causes,
2. differential diagnosis,
3. evaluation, and

4. management of nightmares
5. in adults.

EPIDEMIOLOGY
The true prevalence of nightmares and
nightmare disorder
1. is uncertain
2. due to varying terminology
3. and criteria for defining nightmares
4. across studies.
5. Nonetheless, it is clear that.
6. the occurrence of an occasional
nightmare is common,
7. and that nightmare disorder is much
less common, particularly in adults.

Approximately
1. 50 percent of children
2. report ever having nightmares, and
3. up to 20 percent report having
frequent nightmares.
4. Approximately 85 percent of adults
report having a nightmare
5. at least once a year,
6. and 2 to 6 percent report having
frequent (weekly) nightmares.

A large population-based study of
1. adults over 50 years of age in Korea
demonstrated a

2. 7 percent prevalence of experiencing severe nightmares
3. accompanied by awakenings
4. Nightmare frequency increases with age. with a more than threefold increase in the prevalence of nightmares in adults over 70 years of age 6.3 percent
5. when compared with adults between 50 and 70 years of age 1.8 percent.
6. There was also an association with
    D. suicidal ideation,
    E. depression, and
    F. stress.

A systematic review of
1. more than 100 studies
2. found that nightmares
3. are more commonly reported by females than males
4. during adolescence and young Adulthood.
5. No sex gap was present in younger children or in adults 60 years of age and older.
6. Nightmare content and frequency, like dreams,
7. may also vary across cultures
8. Fear and anxiety related to the COVID-19 pandemic
9. have led to an increase in disrupted sleep and mood symptoms,

10. including nightmares and unwanted dreams.
11. In addition, irregular sleep-wake patterns and
12. disrupted sleep
13. have caused significant emotional and psychological disturbances,
14. in many cases accompanied by more frequent nightmares

CAUSES
1. Nightmares are more prevalent during periods of stress
2. They can emerge in in posttraumatic stress disorder (PTSD),
3. and in association with other psychiatric diagnoses,
4. including depression,
5. dissociative disorders, and
6. borderline personality disorder.
7. Medications most associated with nightmares include those that.
8. affect norepinephrine signaling.
9. dopamine signaling
10. Acetylcholine signaling or
11. gamma-aminobutyric acid (GABA) signaling

Medications
A wide range of medications have been implicated in generating nightmares

1. As an example, beta blocker medications tend to decrease REM sleep, but they are commonly associated with nightmares.
2. Antihypertensives – In one systematic review, beta blockers accounted for one-third of the reports of nightmares as an adverse effect of medications in clinical trials
   A. propranolol,
   B. metoprolol, and
   C. pindolol
   D. Sotalol
   E. Carvedilol
   F. labetalol [
   G. Atenolol
   H. Reserpine h
3. Dopamine agonists – including anti-Parkinson drugs such as
   A. Levodopa,
   B. Pramipexole
   C. Ropinirole
   D. bromocriptine
   E. Amphetamine
   F. methylphenidate.

Antidepressants – during use and withdrawal.
   1. REM sleep, although suppressed,
   2. is delayed until later in the night
   3. and associated with cholinergic rebound.

4. and more intense dream activity.

Antimicrobials –
1. possibly through modulation of sleep-regulating inflammatory cytokines,
2. such as interleukin (IL)-1B,
3. tumor necrosis factor (TNF)-alpha,
4. prostaglandin E2
5. Ciprofloxacin
6. Erythromycin
7. Efavirenz
8. Ganciclovir
9. mefloquine

Antihistaminergic agents,
1. antipsychotic agents,
2. antiseizure drugs,
3. angiotensin-converting enzyme (ACE) inhibitors,
4. and ketamine

Withdrawal from medications —
1. Nightmares commonly occur during withdrawal from
2. GABA-ergic medications or
3. substances such as
4. alcohol,
5. barbiturates, and
6. benzodiazepines (also Paradoxical Agitation during Use)

7. a compensatory increase in REM sleep (ie, REM rebound) that occurs when these medications, which suppress REM sleep, are withdrawn, (rebound nightmares)

Similarly, withdrawal of antidepressant medications, including.
1. Tricyclics,
2. monoamine oxidase inhibitors,
3. selective serotonin reuptake inhibitors (SSRIs), and
4. serotonin-norepinephrine reuptake inhibitors (SNRIs),
5. related to REM rebound.

Idiopathic - Nightmares may occur with increased frequency:
1. during times of stress or
2. emotional instability and
3. may disturb the quality and continuity of sleep.
4. Some have proposed that nightmares may.
5. initially be about the experience of a stressful event but
6. very soon are replaced by the dominant emotion of the event.
7. as a repeating narrative
8. The theme may be fear followed by guilt and other strong emotions.

In a Finnish nationwide twin cohort study, monozygotic twins had more similar rates of nightmares than dizygotic twins, suggesting a genetic propensity.

CLINICAL FEATURES
Nightmares
1. Nightmares are vivid,
2. well-remembered dysphoric dreams
3. that cause awakening.
4. Dream content is typically scary.
5. and vivid,
6. with negative themes
7. that result in disturbed,
8. fragmented sleep.
9. Common themes include.
10. failure and
11. helplessness,
12. physical aggression,
13. accidents, being chased,
14. health-related concerns,
15. death,
16. and interpersonal conflicts

Nightmares are often associated with:
1. a heightened sense of awareness,
2. and increased sympathetic tone as evidenced,
3. by palpitations,
4. increased blood pressure,

5. increased heart rate,
6. sweating,
7. symptoms of anxiety
8. panic upon awakening,
9. recall of vivid, dream content,
10. in contrast with sleep terrors,
11. nightmares generally rise from rapid eye movement (REM) sleep,
12. less commonly out of N2 sleep
13. nightmares most often in the last third of the night,
14. when REM sleep predominates
15. an exception is nightmares associated with
16. post-traumatic stress disorder (PTSD),
17. which are equally likely during N1/N2 and REM sleep and
18. may occur both early and late in the sleep period

Nightmare disorder –
Nightmares that recur with
1. enough frequency
2. and distress
3. to impact nighttime or daytime function
4. may meet criteria for nightmare disorder.

The International Classification of Sleep Disorders, Third Edition, Text Revision (ICSD-3-TR), defines nightmare disorder as follows:

1. Repeated occurrences of extended,
2. extremely dysphoric,
3. and well-remembered dreams
4. that usually involve threats to survival,
5. security, or
6. physical integrity,
7. on awakening from the dysphoric dreams,
8. the person rapidly becomes oriented and alert,
9. the dream experience or sleep disturbance,
10. produced by awakening from it,
11. causes clinically significant distress,
12. or impairment in social,
13. impairment in occupational, or
14. impairment in other important areas of functioning
15. as indicated by the report of at least one of the following:
16. Mood disturbance (eg, persistence of nightmare affect, anxiety, dysphoria)
17. Sleep resistance (eg, bedtime anxiety, fear of sleep or subsequent nightmares),
18. Negative impact on caregiver or

family functioning (eg, nighttime disruption),

19. behavioral problems (eg, bedtime avoidance, fear of the dark),
20. daytime sleepiness,
21. fatigue or low energy,
22. impaired occupational or
23. educational function,
24. or impaired interpersonal or social function,
25. the nighttime symptoms are not attributable to the physiological effects of a substance,
26. and that coexisting mental and medical disorders do not adequately explain the predominant complaint of dysphoric dreams.

Specifiers:
1. During sleep onset,
2. with associated non-sleep disorder, including substance use disorders,
3. with associated other medical condition,
4. with associated other sleep disorder,
5. acute – duration of period of nightmares is ≤1 month,
6. subacute – duration of period of nightmares >1 month, <6 months
7. persistent – duration of period of nightmares is ≥6 months,

8. current severity by the frequency with which the nightmares occur:
9. mild – less than one episode per week on average,
10. moderate – one or more episodes per week but less than nightly.
11. severe – episodes nightly.

Polysomnography
1. Polysomnography (PSG) is not indicated for routine evaluation of nightmares,
2. Nightmares are less likely to occur in the sleep laboratory than in the home environment.
3. PSG may be helpful in selected patients with atypical symptoms to investigate alternative etiologies.

PSG findings in patients with frequent nightmares
1. are inconsistent.
2. one study,
3. using ambulatory PSG
4. found no differences in sleep parameters,
5. between subjects with frequent nightmares and
6. those without,
7. although subjective sleep quality was worse in the nightmare group,

8. and those with nightmares were more likely to complain of insomnia,
9. and those with nightmares were more likely to complain of and daytime dysfunction,
10. during nightmares, measures of autonomic activation have shown an increase in sympathetic activity,
11. nightmare sufferers had reduced sleep efficiencies,
12. increased wakefulness after sleep onset,
13. reduced slow wave sleep, and
14. increased nocturnal awakenings, particularly from N2 sleep,
15. compared with healthy controls.

Limited data suggest that
1. periodic limb movements of sleep (PLMS),
2. may be more frequent in patients with idiopathic nightmares,
3. and nightmares associated with posttraumatic stress disorder (PTSD),
4. compared with healthy controls.

DIFFERENTIAL DIAGNOSIS includes
1. dysphoric dreams ("bad dreams"),
2. other parasomnias, such as rapid eye movement (REM) sleep behavior disorder (RBD) and,

3. sleep terrors,
4. and psychiatric disorders such as
nocturnal panic attack

Clinical features of nightmares that are
helpful in differentiating them from most
other sleep-related phenomena include,
   1. full alertness and upon awakening,
   2. dream recall upon awakening,
   3. occurrence generally later in the
       night when REM is more frequent,
   4. and an absence of motor behavior
       while sleeping.

Dysphoric dreams – Dysphoric dreams, or
"bad dreams," are distinguished from
nightmares.
1. by a lack of awakening from sleep
   like nightmares,
2. bad dreams involve
3. intense negative emotions,
4. most often anxiety and fear,
5. however, the content and intensity of bad
   dreams, tend to be less
6. comprehensively remembered in the
   morning,
7. since awakening is delayed.

REM sleep behavior disorder – RBD should
be suspected.
   1. when dreams or nightmares are

2. associated with motor activity or vocalization,
3. during normal dreaming and REM sleep,
4. most of the major muscle groups are paralyzed (atonic),
5. preventing movement,
6. In RBD, there is loss of normal REM-related atonia,
7. resulting in the ability to move and "act out" dreams,
8. Eszopiclone (Lunesta): The FDA added a boxed warning regarding the potential risk of serious injury from complex sleep behaviors caused by eszopiclone.
9. Zaleplon (Sonata): Like eszopiclone, zaleplon is also associated with parasomnia.
10. Zolpidem (Ambien, Intermezzo): Another medication in the same class, zolpidem, has been linked to sleepwalking and other unusual sleep behaviors[1].

Physical behaviors in RBD
1. range from minor limb movements and groaning,
2. to violent thrashing,
3. punching, and,
4. kicking movements,

5. associated with injury to the patient
6. or bed partner,
7. patients often wake up briefly as a result of the movements and,
8. recall an unpleasant or threatening dream.

RBD is most commonly seen in
1. older adults in association,
2. with neurodegenerative disorders,
3. such as dementia with Lewy bodies,
4. and Parkinson disease,
5. however, symptoms of RBD,
6. may precede cognitive decline,
7. and motor disability,
8. by a decade or more.
9. in younger patients, RBD,
10. may be seen in association with,
11. antidepressant medications,
12. narcolepsy, and,
13. rarely structural brainstem pathology.

Sleep terrors (pavor nocturnus) – Sleep terrors are
1. a disorder of arousal from non-REM (NREM) sleep,
2. in which an individual suddenly sits up in bed, screams,
3. and may flail about,
4. or walk around,

5. there is increased sympathetic nervous system activity,
6. pupillary dilation,
7. sweating, tachycardia,
8. and individuals appear scared and inconsolable,
9. even though they are not clearly aware of their surroundings.

Sleep terrors
1. last a few minutes to as long as 30 to 4 minutes, and,
2. patients are often amnestic for the events,
3. in contrast with nightmares, which occur during REM sleep,
4. sleep terrors usually occur from N3 sleep (delta, slow wave, or deep sleep),
5. and are noted in the early part of the night, when NREM sleep predominates

Sleep terrors caused by taking or withdrawing from many drugs,
1. Prescription Drugs that Cause Nightmares,
2. Antidepressants,
3. Paxil being the primary culprit,
4. Zoloft,
5. Prozac and,
6. Viibryd,

7. Antihistamines,
8. Benadryl,
9. Zyrtec,
10. Claritin,
11. Alegra and,
12. Unisom,
13. Blood pressure medications,
14. Beta-blocker medications,
15. Propranolol,
16. Metoprolol,
17. Atenolol and,
18. Labetalol,
19. Steroids.
20. prednisone and,
21. methylprednisolone
13. Cholesterol medication,
14. Zocor,
15. Pravachol and,
16. Lipitor,
17. Parkinson's medication,
18. Amantadine .
19. Other Drugs that Cause Nightmares
20. withdrawal process can create sleep problems, including unpleasant and vivid dreams,
21. Alcohol,
22. Marijuana,
23. Cocaine,
24. Methamphetamine,
25. and prescription medications

I rely on:
The Recovery Village
Editor Megan Hull
Medically Reviewed by Eric Patterson, LPC
Last Updated: July 12, 2023

Night Terrors
1. are common in children and,
2. are usually benign,
3. in adults, they may be an indicator of,
4. comorbid posttraumatic stress disorder (PTSD),
5. anxiety,
6. or other psychiatric disorders

Nocturnal panic attack –
Patients with nocturnal panic attacks
1. awaken from sleep with a sense of
2. impending doom,
3. sometimes in association with tachycardia,
4. and hyperventilation,
5. the experience is distressing,
6. and is often perceived as a heart attack,
7. due to the intensity of physical symptoms,
8. nocturnal panic attacks are similar,
9. to panic attacks during waking hours,
10. and often lack an identifiable trigger

Unlike nightmares,
1. nocturnal panic attacks,
2. are not usually associated with recall of a dysphoric dream,
3. and the degree of physical hyperarousal,
4. is generally greater than that associated with nightmares.

Hypnopompic/hypnagogic hallucinations –
1. Hallucinations upon awakening (hypnopompic hallucinations)
2. or upon falling asleep (hypnagogic hallucinations),
3. can sometimes be difficult to differentiate from nightmares by history,
4. patients awakening from a nightmare may continue to experience dream content briefly while awake, thereby mimicking a hallucination,
5. patients who have hypnagogic hallucinations can quickly awaken,
6. and believe they had a nightmare.

Hypnopompic hallucinations,
1. are usually visual,
2. but can involve the other senses.,
3. like nightmares, they arise out of REM sleep,

4. Hypnopompic hallucinations are associated with narcolepsy,
5. a disorder characterized by the irrepressible need to sleep,
6. excessive daytime sleepiness,
7. cataplexy, sleep paralysis,
8. and hypnagogic or hypnopompic hallucinations,
9. can also occur idiopathically,
10. or in association with other parasomnias.

Bereavement-related dysphoric dreams –
1. Negatively themed dreams,
2. may occur during or shortly after periods of grief and loss,
3. disrupting sleep,
4. the triggering factor is the death,
5. or loss of a loved one,
6. and the dreams usually occur in the context of a person,
7. who does not routinely have nightmares,
8. dysphoric dreams associated with bereavement,
9. are often self-limited and rarely require specific treatment.

Lucid dreaming –
1. Lucid dreaming occurs,
2. when an individual is aware,

3. that they are dreaming while asleep,
4. when these dreams have negative content,
5. they can resemble a nightmare.

Others:
Nocturnal seizures –
1. rarely, nocturnal seizures,
2. are associated with frightening auras,
3. or ictal imagery,
4. that may mimic a nightmare.
5. in most cases,
6. these symptoms do not occur in isolation,
7. and stereotypical motor activity,
8. and other more typical signs of seizure are present,
9. corroborative history from a bed partner is important,
10. as patients may emphasize the frightening nightmare-like symptom,
11. and not be aware of other seizure manifestations,
12. if suspicion for seizure persists,
13. further evaluation with overnight video-electroencephalography (video-EEG) monitoring can be used to better characterize the spells.

Sleep-related breathing disorder –
1. Arousals or,
2. Awakenings,
3. associated with apneas,
4. and hypopneas,
5. may appear frightening to a bed partner,
6. who may report that the patient is having "scary dreams."
7. similarly, patients,
8. may awaken from a REM-related respiratory event,
9. with choking,
10. or gasping,
11. and either have a perception of a frightening dream,
12. or recount a co-occurring nightmare,
13. for example, about drowning,
14. in such cases,
15. the primary disorder is sleep apnea,
16. and dysphoric dreams are often secondary.

Sleep-related breathing disorder –
1. This can be differentiated from nightmare disorder,
2. by history,
3. and polysomnography

DIAGNOSTIC EVALUATION
1. Nightmare disorder is a clinical diagnosis,
2. a comprehensive clinical evaluation,
3. aims to differentiate nightmares from mimics,
4. identify causes,
5. and contributing factors,
6. and assess the impact on,
7. physical,
8. social,
9. and emotional functioning.

Key the history can include the following:
1. Description of nightmares,
2. including frequency,
3. and duration,
4. assessment of sleep quality,
5. quantity,
6. and any abnormal movements,
7. or behaviors during sleep,
8. potential contributing factors,
9. such as medications,
10. substances,
11. and recent or past stressful life events,
12. history of experiencing a traumatic event,
13. the posttraumatic stress disorder (PTSD) checklist (PCL-5),
14. can be used to screen patients for

PTSD,
15. patients with possible PTSD should receive,
16. a comprehensive psychiatric assessment,
17. signs and symptoms of,
18. relevant comorbidities,
19. including depression,
20. and other psychiatric disorders,
21. patients can be screened for depression with the self-report, two-item Patient Health Questionnaire (PHQ-2),
22. and those who screen positive should be interviewed to diagnos depression.
23. the interview can be facilitated with the self-administered PHQ-9.
24. other commonly used tools include,
25. Beck Depression Inventory,
26. the Structured Clinical Interview for DSM Disorders (SCID),
27. and Hamilton Depression Rating Scale (HAMD)

Adverse consequences on sleep and daytime function.
1. Polysomnography (PSG) is not indicated,
2. to confirm the diagnosis of nightmares or nightmare disorder,
3. PSG may be indicated,

4. if a primary sleep disorder is suspected,
5. such as rapid eye movement (REM),
6. sleep behavior disorder (RBD),
7. or obstructive sleep apnea.

MANAGEMENT
General approach,
1. Nightmares do not always require treatment,
2. Even individuals who meet criteria for nightmare disorder,
3. may find that symptoms resolve over time without specific intervention,
4. or patients who require intervention,
5. we recommend a top-down approach,
6. starting with a broad general evaluation of sleep,
7. and any predisposing trauma,
8. psychiatric disorders or medications,
9. and then moving on to more specific treatment of nightmares when needed.

For patients who require nightmare-specific treatment,
1. clinical guidelines from the American Academy of Sleep Medicine (AASM),
2. endorse both behavioral,
3. and pharmacologic approaches,
4. mong these,

5. imagery rehearsal therapy (IRT),
6. a form of cognitive behavioral therapy (CBT),
7. and prazosin have the largest supporting literature,
8. both have been primarily studied in patients with posttraumatic stress disorder (PTSD),
9. who often have stereotyped,
10. repeated nightmares,
11. and additional symptoms of,
12. hyperarousal,
13. and trial results of prazosin have been inconsistent.

The choice between psychotherapy and medication
1. can be individualized,
2. according to patient preferences,
3. and access to a therapist,
4. in our experience,
5. the majority of chronic persistent nightmares in adults,
6. are related in some way to underlying psychopathology,
7. or past trauma,
8. and we encourage most patients to engage in psychotherapy,
9. prior to or in conjunction with prazosin.

Lifestyle modification and good sleep
hygiene
1. promote good sleep,
2. can help to decrease the frequency
and severity of nightmares,
3. and enhance the overall quality of
sleep,
4. these interventions have,
5. demonstrated efficacy in treating
nightmares,
6. in children and young adults

Although sleep hygiene has not been
studied on its own,
1. in patients with nightmare disorder,
2. it is often a component of studies
involving other treatments,
3. and is a low-cost,
4. low-risk intervention.

Good practice recommendations include
the following:
1. Seek healthy social interaction,
2. to promote emotional stability and
sense of wellbeing,
3. take a warm shower and empty the
bladder prior to sleep,
4. exercise regularly, but not within four
hours of sleep time,
5. avoid greasy fatty foods close to
bedtime

6. do not skip meals, as hunger may influence sleep quality,
7. avoid alcohol close to bedtime,
8. avoid caffeine close to bedtime,
9. and avoid nicotine close to bedtime,
10. keep a consistent schedule for sleep and daytime function,
11. sleep in a comfortable environment,
12. that is conducive to good sleep,
13. appropriate bedding,
14. appropriate temperature,
15. appropriate noise levels,
16. do not watch TV in bed or for an hour before bedtime
17. do not use cell phone in bed or for an hour before bedtime.
18. do not use computers in ebd or for an hour before bedtime,
19. establish a healthy, relaxing bedtime routine,
20. use bed only for sleep and intimacy for sleep conditioning.

Withdrawal of causative medications,
1. when the onset of nightmares is temporally linked to a potentially causative medication,
2. discontinuation of,
3. or gradual decrease in dose will usually result in resolution of the nightmares.

Other etiologies and interventions discussed below should be pursued if nightmares do not resolve with discontinuation of the medication.

Treatment of co-occurring psychiatric disorders,
1. sychiatric assessment and treatment of underlying psychiatric disease are recommended in patients with persistent nightmares,
2. successful treatment of common predisposing conditions such as,
3. stress,
4. anxiety,
5. depression,
6. acute stress disorder (ASD),
7. or PTSD,
8. will often decrease the frequency and severity of nightmare disorder,
9. this may be accomplished in the primary care setting,
10. or through referral to a mental health clinician,
11. depending on the severity of psychiatric symptoms and comfort level of the treating clinician.

However,
1. even with successful treatment of predisposing factors,
2. and co-occurring psychiatric disorders,
3. nightmares can persist and may require specific treatment.

Nightmare-focused psychotherapy
Psychotherapy.
1. to address underlying psychopathology,
2. or past trauma,
3. psychotherapeutic interventions for nightmare disorder,
4. focus on exposure,
5. and stress management,
6. using cognitive and behavioral techniques,
7. which are tailored to assess,
8. identify,
9. modify,
10. and correct distortions of cognition
11. and behavior

A variety of cognitive and behavioral approaches have been studied for patients with nightmare disorder Among these,
1. in most patients,
2. we suggest imagery rehearsal therapy (IRT),

3. a form of cognitive behavioral therapy (CBT),
4. IRT may be most applicable in patients with a recurring nightmare or schema,
5. if IRT is not available,
6. more limited data support other forms of CBT tailored to nightmares.

CBT,
1. is a specialized,
2. short-term,
3. goal-oriented psychotherapeutic approach,
4. that focuses on distorted,
5. or dysfunctional beliefs,
6. thoughts,
7. emotions,
8. and associated behaviors,
9. that influence nightmares,
10. the cognitive component,
11. focuses on distorted thinking,
12. emotions, feelings,
13. and their associated influence on nightmares,
14. and sleep disruption,
15. the behavioral component,
16. is tailored to address,
17. maladaptive behaviors,
18. and actions,
19. that influence poor sleep,

20. and perpetuate nightmares,
21. CBT alone is effective in the treatment of nightmares,
22. although more specialized nightmare-focused treatment variants,
23. like CBT-I,
24. IRT,
25. and exposure,
26. relaxation,
27. and rescripting therapy (ERRT),
28. have improved results.

Imagery rehearsal therapy –
1. IRT,
2. is a specialized,
3. trauma-focused intervention,
4. targeting nightmare disorder,
5. it includes CBT techniques,
6. of initially recalling the nightmare,
7. and negative event,
8. writing it down with details of emotional sensitivity,
9. reading it,
10. and then modifying the theme,
11. the modified story is made more favorable,
12. and the ending of the story line is changed and rewritten,
13. the rewritten dream is then rehearsed,

14. so that the modified, more acceptable dream content will replace the nightmare,
15. if the dream recurs,
16. this technique aims at rescripting,
17. the content,
18. and theme of the nightmare,
19. to decrease the negative emotion from the dream,
20. rendering it bearable,
21. or even favorable to the patient,
22. this technique requires expertise,
23. by the therapist,
24. and practice by the patient for success.

IRT has shown efficacy in patients,
1. with both idiopathic nightmare disorder,
2. as well as trauma-associated nightmare disorder,
3. in a meta-analysis of,
4. 11 randomized trials of IRT alone,
5. or combined with other psychological treatments for nightmares,
6. in patients with PTSD,
7. IRT showed moderate positive effects,
8. on nightmare frequency,
9. and sleep quality,
10. compared with a control condition

Studies assessing the efficacy of IRT with CBT-I
1. have shown mixed results,
2. One trial in 108 war veterans,
3. with PTSD-associated nightmares,
4. found no added benefit of IRT,
5. when combined with CBT-I,
6. compared with CBT-I alone,
7. another smaller RCT of,
8. 42 sexual assault victims,
9. with PTSD,
10. showed benefit with IRT,
11. with no additional benefit when IRT was followed by general CBT.

An important limitation of IRT is,
1. access to qualified practitioners,
2. and studies of online delivery suggest that this model,
3. may be an effective way to expand access,
4. further work needs to be done to standardize the online model,
5. and validate it in different languages.

Cognitive behavioral therapy for insomnia
1. CBT-I
2. is a specialized,
3. and focused cognitive,
4. and behavioral intervention,
5. to manage distorted,

6. and dysfunctional sleep beliefs,
7. and behaviors,
8. the goal is,
9. to help improve quality,
10. and quantity of sleep,
11. with consequent reduction,
12. of frequency,
13. and severity,
14. of nightmares,
15. specifically in individuals,
16. with nightmares,
17. there may be a role for CBT-I,
18. to focus on pre-sleep cognitive arousal,
19. which has been associated,
20. with increased likelihood of nightmares,
21. in trauma survivors

Two randomized trials of veterans with PTSD-related nightmares
1. demonstrated improvement,
2. but in certain areas results were mixed,
3. in one study,
4. veterans who were randomly assigned to CBT-I,
5. over wait-list controls showed significant improvement in Pittsburgh Sleep Quality Index Addendum for PTSD (PSQI-A) scores,

6. which includes a measure of nightmares,
7. but both the CBT-I group,
8. and wait-list controls had a similar decrease in nightmares,
9. on the Clinician-Administered PTSD Scale (CAPS) distressing dreams item,
10. no adverse effects were reported,
11. and the improvements were sustained following treatment,
12. as mentioned in the discussion of IRT,
13. a study of veterans with PTSD-associated nightmares,
14. using both CBT-I and IRT,
15. found CBT-I alone to be as effective in nightmare reduction,
16. as CBT-I combined with the nightmare-specific IRT

Other specialized techniques –
1. More limited data support other forms of CBT tailored for nightmares including,
2. systematic desensitization;
3. progressive deep muscle relaxation training,
4. lucid dreaming therapy,
5. sleep dynamic therapy,
6. self-exposure therapy,
7. ERRT,

8. Hypnosis,
9. and eye movement desensitization and reprocessing (EMDR),
10. the effectiveness of these interventions depends on the expertise of the therapist and the acceptance by the patient.

Pharmacologic therapies
Prazosin,
1. Prazosin,
2. an alpha-1 adrenergic receptor antagonist,
3. is the best studied medication for nightmares,
4. and has been the preferred first-line pharmacotherapy,
5. when medication is deemed necessary,
6. trials of prazosin in patients with PTSD published subsequent to the AASM literature review,
7. have had conflicting results, however

While prazosin
26. remains a reasonable option
27. in patients with nightmares
28. who fail or do not have access to nightmare-focused psychotherapy,
29. further studies are needed

30. to help identify patients who are most likely to respond to prazosin.
31. There is a paucity of data on prazosin
32. and other drugs for patients with idiopathic nightmare disorder.

A 2020 meta-analysis of,
1. seven randomized trials of prazosin in,
2. 528 patients,
3. with PTSD,
4. found that prazosin was,
5. more effective than placebo,
6. at improving nightmares,
7. sleep quality,
8. and illness severity,
9. with moderate,
10. to large effect sizes,
11. that were similar in magnitude to those observed,
12. in controlled trials of IRT or ERRT,
13. most patients were treated,
14. concurrently with psychotherapy,
15. and psychiatric medications,
16. such as,
17. selective serotonin reuptake inhibitors (SSRIs),
18. there was significant between-study heterogeneity,
19. in particular,
20. the largest individual trial in 304 veterans with PTSD,

21. and frequent nightmares,
22. _+_+_
    failed to show benefits of prazosin
    _+_+_+,
23. compared with placebo,
24. in alleviating distressing dreams
25. or improving sleep quality,
26. several limitations of this trial have
    been raised,
27. as potential explanations for the
    discrepant results with prior trials,
28. including a high percentage of
    antidepressant use in both arms,
29. and the exclusion of patients with
    psychosocial instability,
30. which may have excluded more
    severely affected patients,
31. who were most likely to respond to
    adrenergic blockade,
32. this was supported by lower mean
    blood pressures than expected in the
    trial participants,
33. relatively low rates of
    benzodiazepine and alcohol use,
34. low study attrition, and,
35. low use of additional treatments after
    week 10.

Prazosin
1. is typically started at 1 mg at bedtime,
2. and the dose gradually increased

3. at intervals ranging from a few days to weekly as tolerated,
4. the recommended target dose from the Veteran's Administration is,
5. 6 to 10 mg
6. however, efficacy can be seen at lower doses,
7. which may be preferable
8. in low body weight
9. and older individuals.
10. across trials,
11. effective, tolerated mean doses range from 3 to 16 mg,
12. with most studies using final doses in the 10 to 15 mg range,
13. use of a low starting dose and slow titration
14. minimizes the incidence of side effects
15. such as hypotension
16. and syncope
17. treatment effect takes weeks to occur,
18. with most studies showing efficacy by eight weeks.
19. improvement can be seen earlier, however,
20. duration of treatment should be individualized,
21. based on trajectory of response
22. and any adverse events,,

23. once the patient has experienced relief of symptoms
24. for a sustained period of time,
25. one can begin a gradual taper of the medication,
26. with close clinical follow-up.
27. patients who fail to respond to prazosin may benefit from further psychotherapy.

Prazosin's mechanism for action in nightmare disorder,
1. may be its ability to blunt the noradrenergic nervous system,
2. which has been implicated in the hyperarousal state of PTSD,
3. n patients with PTSD,
4. there is evidence for increased sensitivity of the noradrenergic nervous system,
5. and elevated levels of norepinephrine in the cerebrospinal fluid.

Other drugs
1. Data are much more limited for other medications in the treatment of nightmares,
2. as with prazosin,
3. data are drawn primarily from patients with PTSD
4. drugs with possible benefit include,

5. trazodone,
6. gabapentin,
7. clonidine,
8. topiramate,
9. terazosin,
10. atypical antipsychotics such as,
11. olanzapine and,
12. risperidone

One small, blinded cross-over randomized trial suggested that,
    1. nabilone,
    2. a synthetic cannabinoid,
    3. is effective for treating PTSD-associated nightmares,
    4. in military personnel,
    5. but more data are needed,
    6. another small randomized trial found that,
    7. hydroxyzine was more effective than placebo,
    8. for reducing nightmares,
    9. but less effective than prazosin.

Investigational
A prescription smartwatch device called "Nightware,"
    1. was authorized for marketing by the US Food and Drug Administration (FDA),
    2. in 2020 based,

3. on preliminary pilot data showing an improvement in sleep quality,
4. relative to baseline in adults with nightmare disorder,
5. or nightmares associated with PTSD,
6. in a sham-controlled trial,
7. in 65 veterans with trauma-related nightmares,
8. the active device was associated with modest improvements,
9. in subjective sleep quality,
10. that were not statistically significant,
11. if other randomized trials validate efficacy,
12. the device could represent a low-risk nonpharmacologic treatment option.

According to the manufacturer,
1. the device is designed to deliver
2. vibrotactile feedback,
3. during a nightmare episode,
4. in order to produce a micro-arousal,
5. it uses a machine-learning algorithm,
6. to detect changes in sleep physiology,
7. suggestive of nightmares,
8. based on variables such as,
9. heart rate,
10. and motion,
11. in data submitted to the FDA,
12. there were no adverse events related to the device,

13. and there was no evidence of an
increase in daytime sleepiness.

SUMMARY AND RECOMMENDATIONS

Definition
1. Nightmares,
2. are dreams with negative content.,
3. occasional nightmares are common,
4. particularly in children,
5. nightmares decrease in frequency with age,
6. and are more commonly reported by females than males in adulthood,

Nightmare disorder refers to
1. recurring nightmares,
2. with enough frequency,
3. and distress,
4. to impact nighttime,
5. or daytime function

Causes –
In adults,
1. the most common conditions,
2. associated with recurrent nightmares,
3. are acute stress disorder,
4. posttraumatic stress disorder (PTSD),
5. depression,
6. and anxiety,
7. certain medications,

8. and substances,
9. can induce,
10. or exacerbate nightmares,
11. during either treatment,
12. or withdrawal

Differential diagnosis –
The differential diagnosis of nightmares includes,
1. other parasomnias,
2. such as sleep terrors,
3. and rapid eye movement (REM) sleep behavior disorder (RBD),
4. and psychiatric disorders,
5. such as nocturnal panic attack

Diagnostic evaluation –
Nightmare disorder is a clinical diagnosis,
1. a comprehensive clinical evaluation,
2. aims to differentiate nightmares from mimics,
3. identify causes such as a history of trauma,
4. and assess the impact on physical,
5. social, and
6. emotional functioning.

Polysomnography (PSG),
1. not indicated to confirm diagnosis,
2. may be useful to diagnose a primary sleep disorder,

3. such as RBD,
4. or obstructive sleep apnea.

Initial management –
1. lifestyle changes to promote sleep,
2. decrease the frequency and
3. decrease the severity of nightmares,
4. enhance the overall quality of sleep,
5. medications that trigge nightmares,
6. should be reduced or discontinued,
7. psychiatric assessment and treatment,
8. of underlying psychiatric disease is recommended,
9. in patients with persistent nightmares,
10. nightmares often improve with treatment of the primary psychiatric disorder such as,
11. anxiety,
12. depression,
13. PTSD

Severe and chronic nightmares –
Treatments include,
1. psychotherapy,
2. medication,
3. the majority of chronic persistent nightmares in adults are related in some way to,
4. underlying psychopathology,

5. or past trauma, and,
6. encourage patients to engage in psychotherapy prior to or in conjunction with medication.

When psychotherapy is chosen
1. we suggest imagery rehearsal therapy (IRT),
2. 2. a form of cognitive behavioral therapy (CBT) (Grade 2C).
3. IRT may be most applicable in patients with a recurring nightmare or schema
4. if IRT is not available,
5. more limited data support other forms of CBT tailored to nightmares.

When medication is chosen,
1. recommend treatment with prazosin,
2. Prazosin has primarily been studied in patients with,
3. PTSD-associated nightmares,
4. and trials in this population have had conflicting results,
5. if there are co-occurring psychiatric illnesses interventions targeting,
6. anxiety,
7. psychosis,
8. or depression,
9. should used prior to consideration of prazosin.

I rely on:
Nightmares and nightmare disorder in adults
AUTHORS: Rochelle Zak, MDAnoop Karippot, MD, FAASMSECTION EDITOR: Alon Y Avidan, MD, MPHDEPUTY EDITORS: April F Eichler, MD, MPH Michael Friedman, MD
All topics are updated as new evidence becomes available and our peer review process is complete.
Literature review current through: Oct 2023.This topic last updated: Oct 18, 2023.

I am here to do no harm and help if I can.

Thank you for your time and attention.

Be kind and you can be my friend.

William R. Yee M.D., J.D.
Board Certified Psychiatrist.
Practicing Medicine and Psychiatry without interruption since 1972 in Michigan, Indiana, Kentucky, California, Texas, and now in Alaska at your service.

"Pre-Existing text," includes names of symptoms and medical illnesses, medications, people, corporations, law cases, statutes, text of statutes, the titles of articles and books, the content of articles and books cited, FDA Labels and FDA releases and images taken from the internet.

My copyright claim is a claim to the "original text," which is my personal experience as described in the text and my commentary on names of symptoms and medical illnesses, medications, people, corporations, law cases, statutes, text of statutes, the titles of articles and books, the content of articles and books cited, FDA Labels and FDA releases and images taken from the internet.

Cross Tapering Psychotropics
The Long View
William R. Yee M.D., J.D.,

Copyright Applied for Nov. 11, 2023

I want to thank Heather Heidorn for her kind assistance in managing cross tapering of psychotropic medications.

There is no specific cross taper.
Cross tapers are individualized to each patient as each patient is unique in DNA and environmental circumstances.

Also, the taper changes day to day as,
1. circumstances change day to day
2. mental illness does not present a flat line,
3. but undulates over time,
4. whether treated or not.

Unfortunately, mental illness usually relapses, with, or without treatment.

As a result, it is never clear.
Is the patient getting better or worse?
Because of the illness?
Or because of the medication?

Finally, if it takes a long time and an accumulation of medications with polypharmacy,
is the patient getting better because of
1. a spontaneous remission,
2. or because the medications are effective?

This is a very important consideration when the client arrives in a psychiatric hospital on a combination of medications that may include Clozaril.

What is the next medication to try?

What is the next medication to stop?

Is it best to stop all medications?
Establish a baseline?
Then treat knowing that mental illness is being treated and not medication side effects?

Also, how much Tardive Dyskinesia is being masked by the current medications?

The following is based upon my fifty years of clinical experience and fifty years of reading the medical literature, and:
Guidelines for Antipsychotic Medication Switches

https://www.psychdb.com/_media/meds/anti
psychotics/nhs_guidelines_antipsychotic_s
witch.pdf
Approved by HFTDTC: March 2009
Review date: September 2012

Additional references will be added to the
text that follows.

I have reviewed some information and have
decided on a 7-day cross taper due to
   3. The severity of the client's mental
       illness.
   4. The concern for the aggression,
   5. The fact that the client is on
       polypharmacy.

The following is the information I have
acquired.

"There are no published controlled trials on
switching antipsychotics," therefore I must
rely on the client's clinical presentation and
my 50 years of clinical experience and
review of the medical literature since 1968.

The choice of medication is based upon the
available medications, and the client's
choice.

Since I am bound by my oath to do no harm and help if I can, it is the patient's choice, based upon a balancing of the risks and benefits of the medications available.

The client has a choice among "Typical" antipsychotic agents such as a High Potency Haldol or a Low Potency Thorazine, adjuvants such as mood stabilizers including but not limited to lithium, Depakote, and seizure medications such as Dilantin, and carbamazepine.

Clozaril is recommended for treat treatment resistant schizophrenia (TRS).

However, there continues to be questionable data supporting the efficacy advantage of Clozaril.

"For TRS, clozapine appears to be not significantly superior to pooled SGAs in observational studies,
and not significantly superior to other single SGAs in RCTs.
When FGAs/SGAs are pooled, clozapine appears to be superior in improving positive symptoms in RCTs in TRS with a small effect size."
and,

"Clozapine is not superior to SGAs in observational studies, but to most FGAs in RCTs with both small and large effect sizes, except short-term data vs chlorpromazine. There is conflicting evidence regarding the superiority of clozapine vs. pooled SGAs in TRS and clozapine appears inferior to quetiapine with medium effect sizes and aripiprazole medium-term in RCTs with a small effect size.

I refer the reader to:
Efficacy, Acceptability, and Tolerability of Antipsychotics in Treatment-Resistant Schizophrenia: A Network Meta-analysis JAMA Psychiatry. 2016;73(3):199-210.

And:

The failure of Clozapine to be superior to other antipsychotics is a long-standing issue in medical literature.

I refer the reader to:

"Conclusions and relevance: Insufficient evidence exists on which antipsychotic is more efficacious for patients with treatment-resistant schizophrenia, and blinded RCTs-in contrast to unblinded, randomized effectiveness studies-provide little evidence of the superiority of clozapine compared with other second-generation antipsychotics. Future clozapine studies with high doses and patients with extremely treatment-refractory schizophrenia might be most promising to change the current evidence."

See:
Efficacy, Acceptability, and Tolerability of Antipsychotics in Treatment-Resistant Schizophrenia: A Network Meta-analysis JAMA Psychiatry. 2016;73(3):199-210.

Reasons for switching antipsychotic medications include;
1. Persistent positive or negative symptoms,
2. Relapse despite proven compliance,
3. Persistent distressing adverse drug reactions,
4. Change of formulation to assist concordance e.g. switch to depot

Risks Associated with Antipsychotic Switches include, but are not limited to:
1. Relapse,
2. Reduced compliance,
3. Deterioration in physical condition due to adverse drug reactions,
4. Exacerbation of condition due to stress and anxiety from the switch,

5, Potential medication errors during the cross over,

6. Cholinergic rebound, where the second drug has less cholinergic activity.
   A. insomnia,
   B. fatigue,
   C. malaise,
   D. myalgia,
   E. iaphoresis,
   F. rhinitis,
   G. paraesthesia,
   H. GI distress,
   I. headaches and
   J. nightmares.

7. withdrawal dyskinesia, r
8. rebound akathisia,
9. rebound dystonia and
10. Worsening (rebound) tardive dyskinesia may in part be related to
11. cholinergic rebound,
12. Combined adverse drug reactions (ADRs)

Other discontinuation reactions
1. Neuroleptic malignant syndrome (NMS)

Differentiate change in presentation
1. that may be due to reduction in side effects from,
2. increased antipsychotic effect- particularly over first six weeks

If there is no improvement at all after six weeks
1. exclude non- compliance,
2. exclude substance misuse, and
3. exclude inadequate dosage.

Gradually discontinue
1. anticholinergic, or
2. antiakathisia medication,
3. in the second month post switch.

Normalization:
1. of raised prolactin,
2. can take over 3 months,
3. especially important to women,
4. due the implications for advice on
   contraception

Switching Antipsychotic Drugs,
1. Approaches to switching medication
   vary in the rate of change and extent of
   any overlap of agents.
2. Pharmacokinetically and,
3. Pharmacologically
4. ++the lowest risk strategy++
        for switching
   ++ is a drug free interval++.
5. The client must balance the benefits
   against the side effects.

The approaches to switching antipsychotics include but are not limited to the following due to adjustments made to individualize treatments.

1. Drug free interval advantages:
A. Minimal potential for combined adverse drug reactions.
B. Minimal potential for drug interactions,
C. Clarity between side effects of second drug and discontinuation effects from first drug,
D. Anticholinergic /antiakathisia medication can be titrated Independently
E. Reduces potential for additive myelosupression when switching to Clozapine,
F. Low risk of medication errors,

Disadvantages include:
G. Length of time taken
H. High level of monitoring of Individual required, possibly even in-patient care,
 I. Risks of relapse,
 J. Relapse can be misinterpreted as Lack of efficacy of second drug

2. Gradual reduction of drug A followed by starting drug B

Advantages.

A. Low risk of medication error.

B. Straightforward,

Disadvantages

C, Risk of relapse,

D. Potential for combined adverse drug reactions

3. Sudden withdrawal of drug A followed by starting B

Advantages:

A. Appropriate where an acute, severe reaction necessitates abrupt withdrawal e.g. clozapine,

B. Low risk of medication errors,

C. Straightforward

Disadvantages:

D. Risk of relapse especially if discontinuing clozapine,

E. Potential for combined adverse drug reactions,

F. Potential for drug interactions

4. Partial overlap:

Advantages:
A. Good if there is high risk of relapse,
B. Changes are less abrupt,
C. Useful for switch from depot to oral as depot plasma levels decline slowly, and withdrawal reactions have not been reported,
D. Useful for high potency to atypical,
E. Useful where there is potential for cholinergic rebound

Disadvantages:
F. Tapering too quickly can cause inadequate cover,
G. Potential for combined ADRs,
H. Potential for drug interactions,
I. Potential for medication errors,
J. And compliance problems,
K. Incomplete switches can result in
L. polypharmacy

5. Full overlap
Advantages:
A. Useful where relapse prevention is the greatest concern,
B. Low risk of discontinuation effects from first drug,
C. Low risk strategy when changing from depot to oral as allows opportunity to

assess compliance with oral therapy

Disadvantages:
D. Possibility of combined ADRs
E. Potential for drug interactions,
F. Potential for medication errors and
G. Potential for medication compliance
   problems,
H. Incomplete switches can result in
   polypharmacy

Cross Titration Equivalent doses,
1. Lack of agreement exists on
   antipsychotic equivalent doses,
2. Especially for high-potency agents.
3. Sedation can cause confusion over
   equivalence
   e.g. haloperidol is a potent antipsychotic
   with relatively low sedative effects,
4. Some drugs do not have a linear
   relationship between dose and
   antipsychotic effect,
5. Dose frequency with depots may be
   important due to first pass effects,
6. For drugs with wide receptor activity
   conversion tables are inappropriate,
7. as they may result in increased side
   effects and over-sedation,
8. Differences in half-lives may complicate
   calculation,
9. Haloperidol and

10. fluphenazine
11. are particularly problematical
12. and can produce unreliable doses
13. when using conversion calculations,
14. Doses for atypical agents are better defined than with conventional agents,
15. No equivalent doses are appropriate for atypical antipsychotics,
16. Calculations become invalid at the extremes of dose range

British National Formulary (BNF)
High Dose Antipsychotic Therapy

Where more than one antipsychotic is prescribed care should be taken not to exceed to cumulative BNF maximum dose unless the patient has a planned and documented regime of high dose antipsychotic therapy

For patients detained under the Mental Health Act subject to Section 58 approval for consent to treatment, cumulative BNF maximum can only be exceeded if specifically indicated.

More details on high dose antipsychotic therapy are available in the HMHTT High Dose Antipsychotic Therapy Guideline

British National Formulary (BNF)
ANTIPSYCHOTIC MAXIMUM LICENSED
ADULT DOSE i.e. 100%
Oral mg per day

Amisulpride 1200
Aripiprazole 30
Asenapine 20
Cariprazine 6
Chlorpromazine 1000 (500)
Clozapine 900
Flupentixol 18
Haloperidol 20
Lurasidone 148
Olanzapine 20
Quetiapine (Mania & MR preparations)
....800
Quetiapine (Schizophrenia/standard-
release preparations) 750
Paliperidone 12
Risperidone 16 (4)
Sulpiride 2400
Zuclopenthixol Injections mg per day....150
Aripiprazole 30
Haloperidol 20
N.B. TEWV max recommended dose is ...15
Olanzapine 20

Depots / long-acting Injections
Aripiprazole mg per month................... 400
Haloperidol decanoate mg per week 75
Olanzapine mg per week 150

Paliperidone – mg per month.................. 150
Paliperidone – mg every 3 months 525
Paliperidone – mg every 6 months 1000
Risperidone - fortnightly or monthly........25
..............................injection mg per week
Zuclopenthixol decanoate mg per week 600

Table of Antipsychotic Equivalences
Antipsychotic equivalent doses:
Oral Daily dose
(Range, wider range = less certainty)
Chlorpromazine 100mg
Fluphenazine 2mg
„...(1.25 to 5mg)
Levomepromazine ....Not established
Pericyazine 24mg
Perphenazine 8mg
.... (7 to 15mg)
Prochlorperazine 15mg
.... (14 to 25mg)
Promazine 100mg
....(50 to 200mg)
Benperidol 2mg
Trifluoperazine ....5mg (2 to 8mg)
Haloperidol 3mg
....(1 to 5mg)
Flupentixol 2mg
Zuclopenthixol 25mg
                        (25 to 60mg) up to 150mg
Pimozide 2mg (1 to 3mg) Note: long half life

Amisulpride 100mg
....(40 to 150mg)
Sulpiride 200mg
....(200 to 333mg)
Clozapine 100mg
....(30 to 150mg)
Olanzapine ....Not established
Quetiapine ....Not established
Zotepine ....Not established
Risperidone 1.5mg
....(0.5 to 3mg)
Aripiprazole ....Not established

Depot Weekly dose (range)
Fluphenazine ....5 to 10mg
....(1 to 12.5mg)
Pipothiazine 10mg
....(5 to 12.5mg)
Haloperidol 15mg
....(5 to 25mg)
Flupentixol 10mg
....(8 to 20mg)
Zuclopenthixol 100mg
....(40 to 100mg)
Risperidone long acting injection 12.5mg
.................................(as 25mg per fortnight)

Injection Daily dose
...........................Chlorpromazine 25 to 50mg
....intramuscularly (IM)

Haloperidol 1.5mg
intravenously (IV)or intramuscularly (IM)
Ref: Psychotropic Drug Directory 2007
Bazire and information supplied by Drug
Company

Antipsychotic Medication Switches
Switch Issues/problems Recommendation

Oral typical antipsychotic to typical depot
1. Anecdotal evidence uneventful,
2. though there are no formal studies.

Converting to the same drug as depot
1. few problems
2. choosing the equivalent dose
3. Give test dose and
4. start titration of depot to maintenance,
5. withdraw oral medication gradually
6. as depot dose escalates.

Oral haloperidol to depot haloperidol
1. accumulation occurs
2. multiply the total daily dose by 15 to 20
3. to a maximum of 300mg,
4. and administer every 4 weeks.
5. decrease the dose by 25% each month,
6. to the minimum effective dose,
7. elderly or those on <10mg per day orally,
8. should have a dose 10 to 15 times the oral
   dose,

9. every 4 weeks

Oral fluphenazine to depot fluphenazine
1. accumulation occurs
2. approximately 3 weeks of depot therapy,
3. multiply the total daily dose
4. by 1.2 and
5. give as fluphenazine decanoate
6. IM every one to two weeks,
7. ncrease the dose interval to 3 weeks
8. after 4 to 6 weeks of therapy.

From depot to oral
1. cross titration is not necessary when switching from depot to oral.

Commence oral medication on the day the next depot would be due.

From depot to clozapine
1. Increased risk of agranulocytosis.
2. As clozapine is sedative & hypotensive, care is needed.
3. Pharmacokinetic interactions
   are unlikely
4. Start clozapine on day that depot would have been due.
5. Monitor white cell count,
6. Monitor for infection,
7. Monitor for blood pressure,
8. Monitor for level of sedation closely

Switch Issues/problems Recommendation:
1. Typical depot to another typical depot
2. usually no significant problems,
3. direct conversion can be made,
4. by choosing the equivalent dose
5. from the conversion table.
6. Administer the new depot on the date the previous depot was due

Combined oral plus depot to depot alone:
1. unexpectedly relapses,
2. occur more frequently,
3. ncrease the dose of depot
4. before reduction of the oral dose

To clozapine
1. Increased risk of agranulocytosis.
2. sedative
3. hypotension,
4. Pharmacokinetic interactions unlikely
5. Withdraw previous drug and
6. allow a washout period
7. monitor white cell count,
8. monitor signs of infection
9. monitor blood pressure
10. monitor sedation.

From clozapine
1. monitor rapid relapse
2. monitor severe withdrawal symptoms

3. gradually withdraw clozapine
4. simultaneously titrate replacement drug.
5. monitor white cell count,
6. monitor infection,
7. monitor ental state.

From clozapine to olanzapine
1. Reports of severe withdrawal in 2 cases
2. Slow clozapine weaning
3. over 3 or more weeks
4. with anticholinergic cover

From clozapine to quetiapine
1. Have been used together to reduce potential for clozapine induced weight Gain,
2. May be safely switched in any way
3. depending on the reason for switch,
4. problem would be risks associated with
5. relapse due to discontinuation of Clozapine

To oral olanzapine risks include:
1. additive EPS,
2. hypotension and
3. drug interactions unlikely.
4. consider potential for pregnancy if
5. switching from a typical agent
6. Introduce olanzapine and
7. increase dose while at the same time
8. gradually reduce the dose of the first

antipsychotic.

Switch from olanzapine
1. Any method is acceptable,
2. there are no reported problems with
   stopping olanzapine suddenly

Switch Issues/problems Recommendation
To aripiprazole from oral
1. olanzapine,
2. risperidone,
3. thioridazine or
4. haloperidol
5. there were no reported problems
   immediate start at 15mg per day
   and sudden withdrawal of existing agent
8. there were no reported problems
   immediate start at 15mg per day
   followed by withdrawal of
   existing agent over 2 weeks
9. Starting at 10mg per day,
10. and titrating up to 30mg,
11. while withdrawing existing
    antipsychotic over 2 weeks

To oral risperidone
1. Hypotensive- may result in additive
   hypotension with low potency drugs.
2. Gradually increase dose over ≥ 3 days
   to 4-6mg per day,
3. a sudden switch may be successful in

60% of individuals.

However, one review recommended
1. avoiding a sudden switch from risperidone
2. Few problems
3. but there is potential for NMS,
4. increased prolactin and
5. additive EPS
6. if switching to phenothiazines
7. if switching to D2 blockers

From risperidone to olanzapine
1. For elderly/frail patients
2. gradually discontinue and
3. then gradually introduce
4. of three methods
5. the most successful method
6. was starting 10mg daily of olanzapine
7. and then gradually reducing
8. and stopping risperidone

Switch Issues/problems Recommendation
Haloperidol to risperidone
1. Neuroleptic Malignant Syndrome (NMS)
2. Caution- monitor closely for signs of NMS

From quetiapine
1. Few problems, any method may be considered to risperidone long

acting injection (RLA).

2. Therapeutic levels are not reached until week 4

3. and do not become optimal until

5 to 6 weeks after starting.

4. Oral cover is essential

5. there is potential for polypharmacy

6. Assess response to oral risperidone

7. before initiation, as recommended by SPC.

8. Oral therapy should continue for 3 to 4 weeks before being gradually reduced.

9. Doses of RLA above 25mg per 2 weeks are rarely necessary and

10. associated with a high incidence of ADR without antipsychotic gain.

11. Typical depot to RLA As 'To risperidone long-acting injection (RLA)'

12. Assess response to oral risperidone before initiation, as recommended by SPC.

13. Manufacturer recommends starting RLA one week before the last the last fortnightly injection

14. with oral therapy if relapse risk high.

15. Alternative strategy- switch on date depot due and supplement with oral risperidone for 3 to 4 weeks.

From RLA to typical depot
1. The manufacturer recommends 8 weeks after the last risperidone long-acting injection before commencing an alternative depot.
2. Plasma levels remain at steady state for 5 weeks after the last injection.
3. Where specific recommendations are found in the literature, they are often based on single case reports or data derived from a limited number of cases.
4. The potential for inter-individual variation should always be considered.

I have heard of unpublished reports of 10,000mg of Chlorpromazine.
However, I could only find published doses of 5,000mg of Chlorpromazine.

Massive doses of antipsychotic medications have failed and are not considered the best practice.

I refer the reader to:

"While most investigators report prescribing daily dosages of 300 to 800 mg in schizophrenia, some have used as much as 5,000 mg daily."

Massive Doses of Chlorpromazine: Effectiveness in Controlling Psychotic Behavior.

APPLETON W. Arch Gen Psychiatry. 1963;9(6):586–592. doi:10.1001/archpsyc.1963.01720180058008

In 2015 and 2016 I received CME's for treating clients with high doses of Medications.

Rational Use of High Dose Antipsychotics for Aggressive Patients
December 14, 2016
WebEx from DSH-Vacaville
And is awarded 1.0 AMA PRA Category 1 Credit(s) TM

Agonist Antipsychotics Work at 83%-98% D2 Occupancy

Conclusion: For a small subset of patients, the EPS threshold may never be reached. Based on this observation, there is probably a point of futility for most antipsychotics beyond which the likelihood of response is virtually nil:
• Haloperidol > 30 ng/mL
• Fluphenazine > 4.0 ng/mL
• Olanzapine > 200 ng/mL"

"The Point of Futility
Meyer JM. A rational approach to employing high plasma levels of antipsychotics for violence associated with schizophrenia: case vignettes. CNS Spectrums 2014; in press

"This article enumerates rational guidelines for employing high plasma level strategies, emphasizing the appropriate interpretation of, and reaction to high plasma antipsychotic levels in these treatment resistant patients, and the need to push treatment to the limits of tolerability or clinical response."

Meyer JM. A rational approach to employing high plasma levels of antipsychotics for violence associated with schizophrenia: case vignettes. CNS Spectr. 2014 Oct;19(5):432-8. doi: 10.1017/S1092852914000236. Epub 2014 May 27. PMID: 24865765.

A rational approach to employing high plasma levels of antipsychotics for violence associated with schizophrenia: case vignettes.
Jonathan M. Meyer
CNS Spectrums / First View Article / August 2014, pp 1 - 7

DOI: 10.1017/S1092852914000236, Published online: 27 May 2014
Link to this article:
http://journals.cambridge.org/abstract_S109 2852914000236

Understanding D2 Blockade and Plasma Antipsychotic Levels

Jonathan M. Meyer, M.D.
Psychopharmacology Resource Network
California Department of State Hospitals
Assistant Clinical Professor of Psychiatry
University of California, San Diego

Maximum daily dosages and estimated therapeutic ranges for SGAs- Estimated therapeutic serum concentration range.

Aripiprazole ....30 ....150 to 350 ng/mLb
Asenapine ......20 ....1 to 5 ng/mLb
Brexpiprazole ...4 ....40 to 140 ng/mLb
Cariprazine .....6 ....10 to 20 ng/mLb
lozapine ....900 ....350 to 600 ng/mLb
Iloperidone .....24 ....5 to 10 ng/mLb
Lumateperone 42 ....Not well established
Lurasidone ....160 ....15 to 40 ng/mLb
Olanzapine ......20 ....20 to 80 ng/mLb
Paliperidone ....12 ....20 to 60 ng/mLb
Quetiapine .....800 ....100 to 500 ng/mLb
Risperidone ....16.....................0 to 60 ng/mLb
Ziprasidone ....200 ....50 to 200 ng/mLb

"In light of safety concerns and a lack of high quality evidence for high-dose antipsychotic therapy, alternative solutions for inadequate response to treatment should be considered. Underlying causes of poor response should be addressed."

Efficacy and safety of high-dose antipsychotic therapy
Brittany Finocchio, PharmD, BCPP
Current Psychiatry Vol. 20, No. 6
 June 2021
ED95 95% effective dose for 95% NNT not stated:
1. Oral aripiprazole.
    ED95 12 mg/day
2. Aripiprazole LAI (lauroxil).
    The ED95 was 463 mg every 4 weeks.
3. Asenapine.
    ED95 was 15 mg/day
4. Brexpiprazole.
    ED95 was 3.4 mg/day
5. Cariprazine.
    ED95 was 7.6 mg/day
6. Clozapine.
    ED95 was 567 mg/day.
7. Haloperidol.
    ED95 was 6.3 mg/day
8. Iloperidone.
    ED95 was 20.1 mg/day.

9. Lurasidone.
   ED95 was 147 mg/day.
10. Oral olanzapine for patients with positive symptoms.
    ED95 was 15.1 mg/day.
11. Oral olanzapine for patients with predominant negative symptoms.
    ED95 was 6.5 mg/day
12. Olanzapine LAI.
    ED95 was 277 mg every 2 weeks.
13, Oral paliperidone.
    ED95 was 13.4 mg/day.
14. Paliperidone LAI.
    ED95 was 120 mg every 4 weeks.
15. Quetiapine.
    ED95 was 482 mg/day,
16. Oral risperidone.
    ED95 was 6.3 mg/day
17. Risperidone LAI.
    ED95 was 37 mg every 2 weeks.
18. Sertindole.
    ED95 was 22.5 mg/day,
19. Ziprasidone.
    ED95 was 186 mg/day

See:

Dose-Response Meta-Analysis of Antipsychotic Drugs for Acute Schizophrenia
Stefan Leucht, M.D., Alessio Crippa, Ph.D., Spyridon Siafis, M.D., Maxine X. Patel, M.D., Nicola Orsini, Ph.D., John M. Davis, M.D.

After seven years,
Patients who stop their medications after a psychotic episode,
1. have a functional recovery rate: of 40.4%.
Patients who continued maintenance medications for seven years,
2. had a functional recovery of 17.6 percent.

Although medications can help resolve an acute psychotic episode,
continuing the medications interferes with a functional recovery.

I rely on:
Post by Former NIMH Director Thomas Insel: Antipsychotics: Taking the Long View
By Thomas Insel on August 28, 2013
Published Online:16 Dec 2019https://doi.org/10.1176/appi.ajp.2019.190 10034

Raising antipsychotics above D2 saturation of 65% does not give additional benefits.

1. There no relationship between saturation,
2. "above 65% and clinical response."
3. That is raising saturation above 65% did not appear to yield additional benefit.
4. raising D2 saturation above 65%

increased prolactin levels and
extrapyramidal side effects.
5. 2.5mg a day of Haldol achieved 65% to
   75% D2 occupancy.
6. They recommended a starting dose of
   two or three milligrams a day.

I rely on:
Relationship Between Dopamine D 2
Occupancy, Clinical Response, and Side
Effects: A Double-Blind PET Study of First-
Episode Schizophrenia
Shitij Kapur, M.D., Ph.D., F.R.C.P.C., Robert
Zipursky, M.D., F.R.C.P.C., Corey Jones,
B.A., Gary Remington, M.D., Ph.D.,
F.R.C.P.C., and Sylvain Houle, M.D., Ph.D.,
F.R.C.P.C. Am J Psychiatry 157:4, April 2000

I am here to do no harm and help if I can.

Thank you for your time and attention.

Be kind and you can be my friend.

William R. Yee M.D., J.D.
Board Certified Psychiatrist.
Practicing Medicine and Psychiatry
without interruption since 1972 in
Michigan, Indiana, Kentucky, California,
Texas, and now in Alaska at your service.

"Pre-Existing text," includes names of Symptoms and medical illnesses, medications, people, corporations, law cases, statutes, text of statutes, the titles of articles and books, the content of articles and books cited.

My copyright claim is a clam to the "original text," which is my personal experiences as described in the text above and my commentary on the names of Symptoms and medical illnesses, medications, people, corporations, law cases, statutes, text of statutes, the titles of articles and books, the content of articles and books cited.

www.ingramcontent.com/pod-product-compliance
Lightning Source LLC
Chambersburg PA
CBHW022116170526
45157CB00004B/1665